This Health Hazard Evaluation (HHE) report and any recommendations made herein are for the specific facility evaluated and may not be universally applicable. Any recommendations made are not to be considered as final statements of NIOSH policy or of any agency or individual involved. Additional HHE reports are available at http://www.cdc.gov/niosh/hhe/

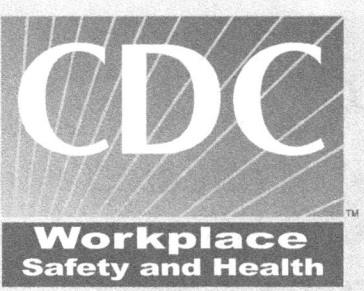

I0426399

Evaluation of Exposures to Healthcare Personnel from Cisplatin during a Mock Interperitoneal Operation

James Couch MS, CIH, REHS/RS
Gregory Burr, CIH

Health Hazard Evaluation Report
HETA 2009-0121-3106
University Medical Center
Las Vegas, Nevada
March 2010

Department of Health and Human Services
Centers for Disease Control and Prevention

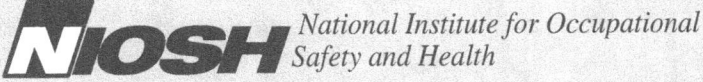 National Institute for Occupational Safety and Health

The employer shall post a copy of this report for a period of 30 calendar days at or near the workplace(s) of affected employees. The employer shall take steps to insure that the posted determinations are not altered, defaced, or covered by other material during such period. [37 FR 23640, November 7, 1972, as amended at 45 FR 2653, January 14, 1980].

CONTENTS

ABBREVIATIONS

µg	Microgram
µg/m^3	Micrograms per cubic meter
ACGIH®	American Conference of Governmental Industrial Hygienists
AIHA	American Industrial Hygiene Association
BEI®	Biological exposure index
CFR	Code of Federal Regulations
cm	Centimeter
GA	General area
HHE	Health hazard evaluation
IARC	International Agency for Research on Cancer
ICP-MS	Inductively coupled plasma mass spectrometry
IV	Intravenous
LOD	Limit of detection
LOQ	Limit of quantification
MDC	Minimum detectable concentration
mL	Milliliter
NAICS	North American Industry Classification System
NIOSH	National Institute for Occupational Safety and Health
OEL	Occupational exposure limit
OSHA	Occupational Safety and Health Administration
PBZ	Personal breathing zone
PEL	Permissible exposure limit
PPE	Personal protective equipment
REL	Recommended exposure limit
STEL	Short-term exposure limit
TLV®	Threshold limit value
TWA	Time-weighted average
UMC	University Medical Center
WEEL	Workplace environmental exposure level

HIGHLIGHTS OF THE NIOSH HEALTH HAZARD EVALUATION

The National Institute for Occupational Safety and Health (NIOSH) received a request for a health hazard evaluation from the management of the University Medical Center in Las Vegas, Nevada. The request concerned potential healthcare personnel exposures to cisplatin during a mock interperitoneal procedure.

What NIOSH Did

- We evaluated the facility on May 11–12, 2009.

- We took wipe samples and area and personal breathing zone air samples for cisplatin. Samples were taken during the pharmacy preparation, a mock interperitoneal procedure, cleaning of the operation room, and sterilization of the surgical equipment.

- We checked to see if the gloves worn by the employees protected them from cisplatin. We did this by asking employees to wear cotton gloves beneath their chemotherapy-approved gloves, which were then analyzed for cisplatin.

What NIOSH Found

- Cisplatin was not found in any of the general area or personal breathing zone air samples.

- Cisplatin was found on one of 15 wipe samples collected. This wipe sample was taken on the operating room floor after the mock interperitoneal procedure before the room was cleaned. No cisplatin was found at this same location after the operating room was sanitized.

- Cisplatin was not found on any of the cotton glove samples.

What Managers Can Do

- Require employees to wear two pairs of chemotherapy protective gloves.

- Train employees on the importance of minimizing splashes and spills of cisplatin solution. Such incidents should be promptly cleaned up and materials properly disposed in chemotherapy receptacles.

What Employees Can Do

- Follow the health and safety measures put into action by hospital management such as wearing two pairs of chemotherapy-approved gloves.

- Place cisplatin-contaminated equipment and materials in appropriate receptacles for either disposal or sterilization.

- Avoid splashing or spilling cisplatin during the interperitoneal procedure. Promptly clean up spills if they occur.

SUMMARY

NIOSH investigators evaluated potential cisplatin exposures before, during, and after a mock interperitoneal procedure. We detected no cisplatin in any air or hand-wipe samples. We did detect cisplatin in one surface wipe sample collected on the operating room floor after the mock procedure before the room was sanitized. No cisplatin was found at this same location after the room was sanitized. We recommend that surgical staff continue to use chemotherapy-approved gloves and handle the cisplatin solution carefully.

On March 24, 2009, NIOSH received a management request for an HHE at the UMC, in Las Vegas, Nevada. The HHE request was submitted because a new medical procedure was being proposed, and some hospital staff were concerned about potential exposures to cisplatin.

On May 11–12, 2009, we visited UMC to evaluate potential exposures to cisplatin during a mock demonstration of the new interperitoneal procedure. We collected GA and PBZ air samples and wipe samples for cisplatin. We evaluated the effectiveness of the chemotherapy-approved gloves worn by the employees by asking employees to wear cotton gloves beneath their chemotherapy-approved gloves. These cotton glove samples were then analyzed for cisplatin.

No cisplatin was detected in any GA air samples (MDC = 0.016 $\mu g/m^3$), personal breathing zone air samples (MDC = 0.058 $\mu g/m^3$), or cotton glove samples (LOD = 0.009 μg/sample). Cisplatin was detected above the LOQ of 0.031 μg/sample on one of the 15 wipe samples taken. This surface wipe sample was taken on the operating room floor near the surgical technician. No cisplatin was detected in surface wipe samples taken in the same area both prior to the interperitoneal procedure and after the room was sanitized (LOD = 0.007 μg/sample). This suggests that the UMC environmental services staff effectively removed any cisplatin contamination following the interperitoneal procedure.

We recommend that employees continue to double-glove by wearing two pairs of chemotherapy-protective gloves. We also recommend that management stress to employees the importance of minimizing splashes and spills. Cisplatin solution splashes or spills should be cleaned up promptly with proper disposal in chemotherapy receptacles.

Keywords: NAICS 622110 (General Medical and Surgical Hospitals), cisplatin, antineoplastic drugs, air samples, surface wipe samples, glove samples

On March 24, 2009, NIOSH received a management request for an HHE at the UMC, in Las Vegas, Nevada. The UMC opened in 1931 and employs more than 4,000 employees. The HHE request was submitted because a new procedure was being proposed, and potential exposures to cisplatin concerned some hospital staff. Cisplatin is an inorganic, antineoplastic oncology drug approved by the Federal Drug Administration for treatment of cancers such as bladder and ovarian cancer [NCI 2009]. Cisplatin has been categorized as a probable human carcinogen by the IARC [IARC 2004].

On May 11–12, 2009, NIOSH investigators visited UMC to evaluate potential exposure to cisplatin during a mock demonstration of a proposed new interperitoneal procedure. We met with management and employee representatives and observed work processes/practices and workplace conditions. During the opening meeting we discussed the nature of the HHE and the types of sampling to be performed to evaluate cisplatin exposures. Representatives from the Service Employees International Union and hospital management were present during the meeting and provided input into other areas of concern within the hospital. We collected air, wipe, and cotton glove samples and analyzed them for cisplatin. A closing meeting was held on May 12, 2009, with UMC management, employees, and the Service Employees International Union to summarize site visit activities and provide preliminary findings. This was followed up with a letter dated August 4, 2009, that provided a preliminary summary and recommendations (sample results were not available at the time of the letter).

Process Description

Various UMC departments and personnel are potentially exposed to cisplatin during the preparation of the cisplatin solution by hospital pharmacy staff; the use of the cisplatin during the interperitoneal procedure; and the subsequent sanitization of the operating room, sterilization of medical equipment, and disposal of the potentially contaminated materials following completion of the interperitoneal procedure. To prepare the desired concentration, an employee in the hospital pharmacy injects cisplatin into an IV bag containing a saline solution. The pharmacy employee dons PPE (surgical mask, two pairs of chemotherapy protective gloves, chemotherapy protective covering, and hairnet) and performs the procedure in a ventilated laboratory hood. A nurse delivers the IV bag to the operating room.

The interperitoneal procedure is performed in an operating room by a surgeon, surgical technician, anesthesiologist, and nurses. During the mock procedure, all employees in the operating room except the surgeon wore powered air purifying respirators with high efficiency particulate air filters, two pairs of chemotherapy protective gloves, a chemotherapy protective covering over scrubs, and disposable coverings over shoes. The surgeon, a nonhospital employee, chose a surgical mask as his only PPE during the procedure. Powered air purifying respirators with a high efficiency filter were chosen by the hospital management because the procedure was new to the hospital and because of the uncertainty about the airborne exposure hazard. The cisplatin solution is emptied by tubing from the IV bag directly into an open body cavity where the surgeon manipulates the target organs in an effort to increase cisplatin absorption. The mock interperitoneal procedure used a metal pan (room temperature) to simulate the open body cavity. The dwell time of the cisplatin solution ranges from 20–90 minutes based upon the treatment protocol. At the end of the desired dwell time the cisplatin solution is suctioned out of the body cavity into a closed container. The body cavity is then closed and the patient is removed to recovery. Disposable items are placed into waste receptacles labeled as chemotherapy waste.

Surgical equipment and other items that may be reused are packaged in a yellow chemotherapy waste bag and sent to the Sterile Processing department. Upon receipt in Sterile Processing, the equipment is rinsed with water to remove gross contamination, washed with a 10% bleach/water solution, and then placed into a 1% sodium thiosulfate/water solution (to neutralize any residual chlorine).

Environmental Services personnel sanitize the operating room by wiping down the walls, floors, and any other accessible surfaces with a 10% bleach solution and then again with a sodium thiosulfate solution to neutralize any residual chlorine. All disposable material is placed into waste receptacles labeled as chemotherapy waste. Environmental Service employees wore a powered air purifying respirator with a high efficiency particulate filter, two pairs of chemotherapy protective gloves, a chemotherapy protective covering over scrubs, and disposable coverings over shoes.

ASSESSMENT

On May 11–12, 2009, we collected air, wipe, and cotton glove samples and analyzed them for cisplatin. The mock interperitoneal procedure introduced a 5% cisplatin solution (100 mL of cisplatin in 1,900 mL of saline) into a metal pan. Neither the cisplatin solution nor the metal pan was heated to simulate the body temperature of the open cavity during the actual procedure. The surgeon allowed the 2,000 mL cisplatin solution to dwell in the metal pan for 20–25 minutes while intermittently manipulating the solution with his gloved hands to simulate massaging the solution into the target organs. The cisplatin solution was then suctioned out of the metal pan. All disposable material was then packaged into chemotherapy bags and placed in the corner of the room to be removed by Environmental Services. All reusable equipment was packaged in chemotherapy bags and sent to Sterile Processing.

General area air samples were taken using a high volume sample pump operating at 15 liters per minute. PBZ air samples were collected using air sampling pumps operating at 4 liters per minute. All of the air samples were taken for the duration of the mock interperitoneal procedure (approximately 45 minutes). Figure 1 shows the locations of GA and PBZ samples along with basic dimensions of the operating room. Figure 2 shows a GA and PBZ sample being collected during the mock interperitoneal procedure.

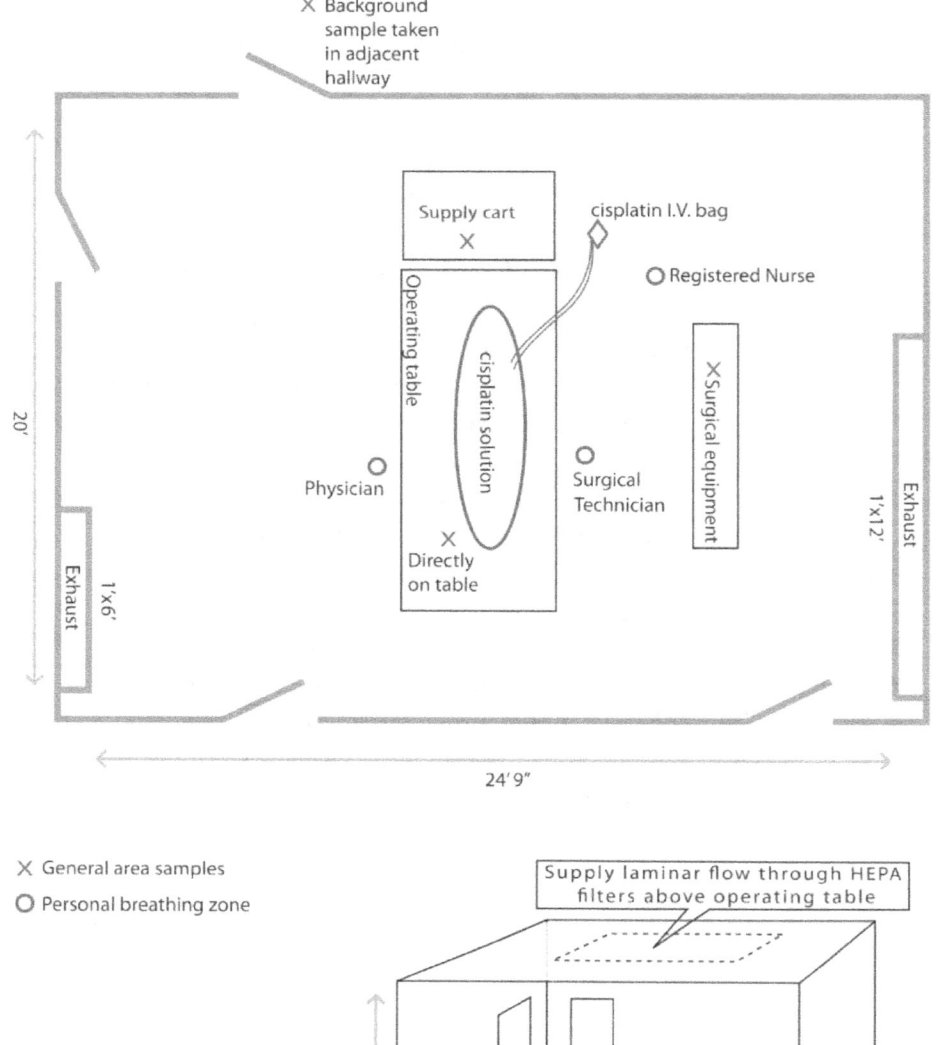

Figure 1. Operating Room 9 dimensions, orientation of air and wipe samples, location of ventilation supply and exhaust, and background sample location outside the operating room.

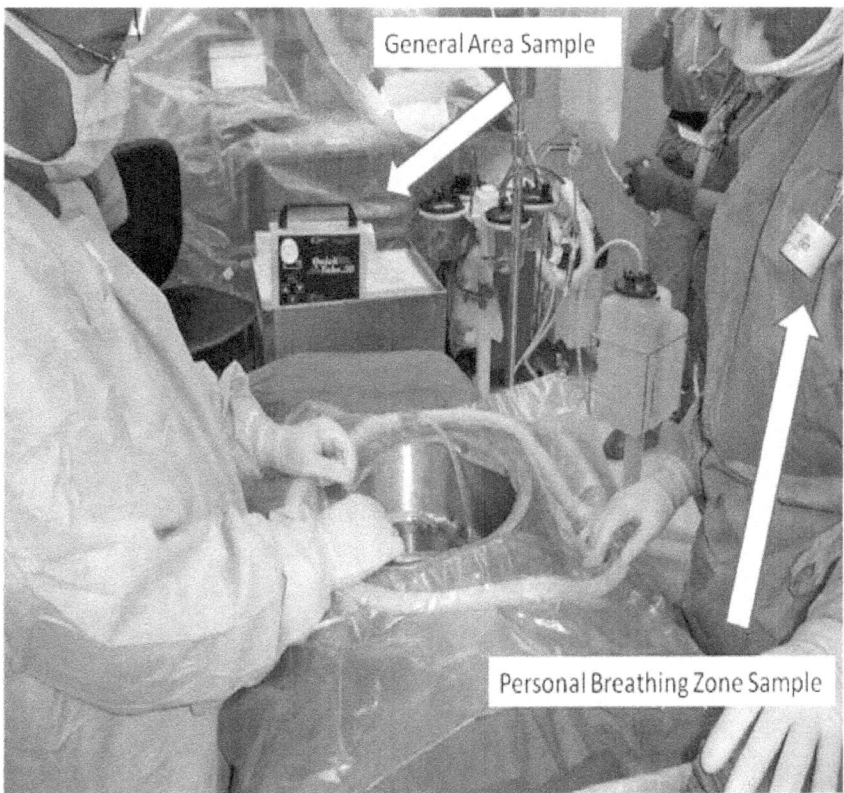

Figure 2. General area and personal breathing zone samples collected during the cisplatin interperitoneal mock procedure.

Surface wipe samples were taken using Alpha Texwipe® swabs moistened with deionized water. A 10 cm x 10 cm square template was used to determine a 100 cm² sampling area. The surface wipe samples were collected on the floor in three locations before the mock procedure, immediately after the mock procedure, and after the room was sanitized. Figure 3 shows the location of the surface wipe samples. Figure 4 shows a NIOSH investigator collecting a surface wipe sample.

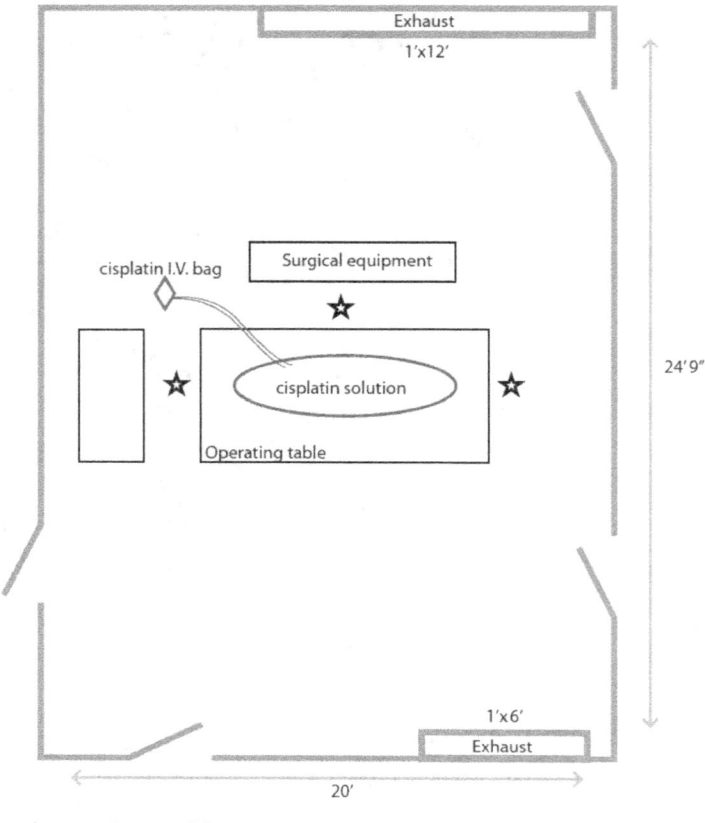

Figure 3. Diagram of Operating Room 9 showing the location of the wipe samples and room dimensions.

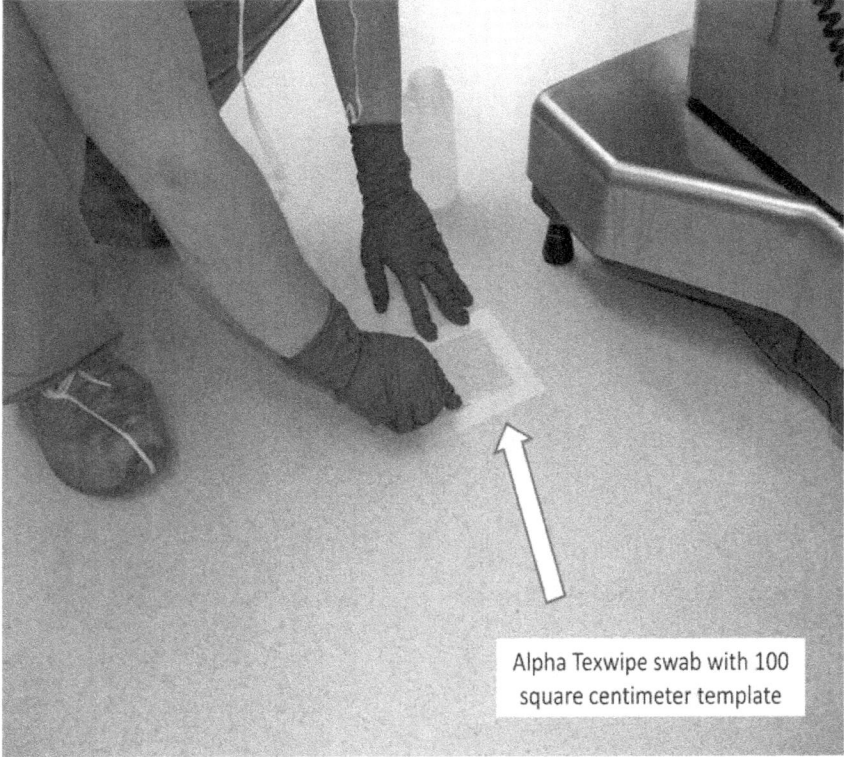

Alpha Texwipe swab with 100
square centimeter template

Figure 4. Collection of wipe sample with Alpha Texwipe swabs with a 100 cm^2 template.

To evaluate potential dermal exposure we asked employees to wear 100% cotton gloves (Lab Safety Supply, Janesville, Wisconsin) beneath their Biogel® latex gloves or nitrile chemotherapy protective gloves. The cotton gloves were then collected and analyzed for cisplatin to evaluate potential dermal exposure from permeation or leakage through the gloves or contamination when the employee donned or doffed them. Wearing sterile gloves, we removed the cotton gloves from the employees after they had removed their outer chemotherapy protective gloves. Figure 5 shows a NIOSH investigator removing the cotton glove sample after the employee had already removed the nitrile chemotherapy protective gloves. The cotton gloves were worn beneath chemotherapy protective gloves so NIOSH investigators could evaluate permeation by cisplatin and hand contamination from donning/doffing the gloves.

All of these sample media were analyzed for cisplatin (as platinum) by ICP/MS. More information on the air, surface, and glove sample collection and analysis is provided in Appendix A. Information on OELs and health effects for cisplatin are discussed in Appendix B.

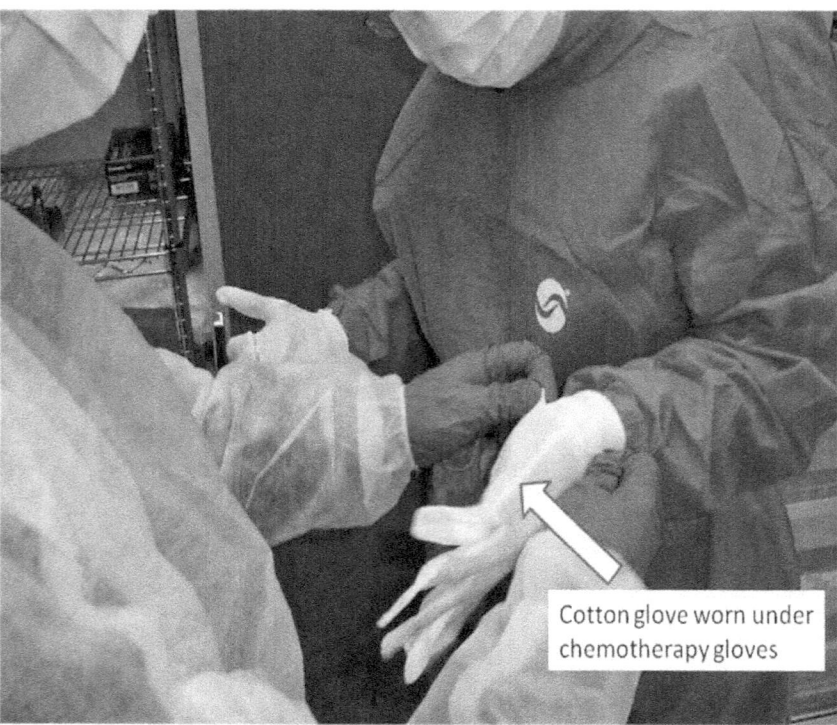

Cotton glove worn under chemotherapy gloves

Figure 5. NIOSH investigator collecting a cotton glove sample.

RESULTS

Air samples (GA and PBZ) were collected in the Inpatient Pharmacy, the operating room (before, during, and after the mock procedure, and then during the operating room sanitization), and Sterile Processing. Airborne cisplatin was not detected; concentrations were below the MDC (0.016 µg/m³ for the GA air samples and 0.058 µg/m³ for the PBZ air samples). The air sampling locations and results are presented in Appendix C, Table C1.

Surface wipe samples were taken in the Inpatient Pharmacy, the operating room, Sterile Processing, and from the hands of two employees. All wipe sample results are shown in Appendix C, Table C2. Cisplatin was detected in one surface wipe sample that was collected on the floor after the mock interperitoneal procedure but before the operating room was sanitized. Figure 3 illustrates the location of the wipe samples taken on the floor of the operating room.

No cisplatin was detected (LOD = 0.009 μg of cisplatin per sample) on any of the cotton gloves worn beneath the chemotherapy protective gloves. As shown in Appendix C, Table C3, cotton glove samples were worn by employees in the Inpatient Pharmacy, during the mock interperitoneal procedure, and during room sanitization and equipment sterilization.

DISCUSSION

Cisplatin was detected on only one surface wipe sample. Because no cisplatin was detected at this sample location before the mock interperitoneal procedure and after the room was sanitized, this result suggests that the floor became contaminated with cisplatin during the mock interperitoneal procedure but was effectively removed during the sanitization process. It also shows the potential for chemotherapy drug contamination of the floor that could contribute to employee exposure to chemotherapy drugs.

Cisplatin was not detected on any air samples. This is not unexpected because cisplatin in a saline solution has a low vapor pressure (approximate to water), meaning that it will not readily volatilize at room temperature [Bedford Laboratories 2009]. Additionally, in the mock interperitoneal procedure the cisplatin solution was gently hand-stirred but not agitated, further lessening the chance that an airborne mist or aerosol could be created. There are no occupational exposure limits specifically for cisplatin in the air or on surfaces.

Cisplatin was not detected on any cotton gloves worn beneath the chemotherapy protective gloves that are normally worn when handling chemotherapy drugs. These results suggest that the chemotherapy protective gloves were protective against permeability of cisplatin during this mock procedure and that the glove donning and doffing procedures followed by the UMC staff did not result in skin contact with cisplatin.

Our findings only apply to this mock procedure. Additional monitoring during an actual procedure is needed because of the variations listed below or if any substantial changes are made to the procedure. Potential exposures to hospital staff during an actual procedure may differ based upon the following:

- Absorption of platinum from the cisplatin solution into the patient's body

DISCUSSION
(CONTINUED)

- Placing surgical instruments directly into the aluminum basin, an action that would not have occurred during an actual procedure

- Amount of manipulation of the cisplatin solution by the surgeon

- Temperature of the aluminum basin holding the cisplatin solution being lower than the temperature of a body cavity, which may lead to a difference in volatilization of materials

CONCLUSIONS

Based on our observations and review of standard operating procedures, UMC employees are potentially exposed to cisplatin when mixing this drug in the pharmacy, administering it during the mock interperitoneal procedure, sanitizing the operating room following cisplatin use, and cleaning and sterilizing the medical instruments. However, the use of chemotherapy protective gloves was effective in preventing dermal exposure to cisplatin during all of these activities. Results from the wipe sampling demonstrated that the mock interperitoneal procedure resulted in limited contamination with cisplatin, and that sanitation procedures effectively removed this contamination. Results from air sampling indicate that no detectable airborne exposure to cisplatin occurred during preparation of the cisplatin solution, during the mock interperitoneal procedure, or during room sanitizing or instrument sterilization.

RECOMMENDATIONS

Based on our findings we encourage UMC to use the following recommendations to develop an action plan based, if possible, on the hierarchy of controls approach (Appendix B: Occupational Exposure Limits and Health Effects). This approach groups actions by their likely effectiveness in reducing or removing hazards. In most cases, the preferred approach is to eliminate hazardous materials or processes and install engineering controls to reduce exposure or shield employees. Until such controls are in place, or if they are not effective or feasible, administrative measures and/or personal protective equipment may be needed.

RECOMMENDATIONS
(CONTINUED)

Administrative Controls

Administrative controls are management-dictated work practices and policies to reduce or prevent exposures to workplace hazards. The effectiveness of administrative changes in work practices for controlling workplace hazards depends on management commitment and employee acceptance. Regular monitoring and reinforcement are necessary to ensure that control policies and procedures are not circumvented in the name of convenience or production. The following administrative controls are recommended to reduce the employees' personal exposures to the cisplatin.

1. Minimize splashing and spilling the cisplatin solution by gently manipulating the solution within the cavity and at target organ(s) when possible.

2. Promptly clean and dispose of any cisplatin solution spilled during the procedure.

3. Continue to use two pairs of chemotherapy protective gloves when handling cisplatin and other chemotherapy drugs.

4. Continue to wear chemotherapy protective gowns made of polyethylene-coated polypropylene.

5. Institute an awareness training program that includes management and employees learning more about cisplatin and other antineoplastic drugs. The following websites provide more information on occupational and environmental exposures, scientific research, and health concerns related to antineoplastic drugs:

   - NIOSH: http://www.cdc.gov/niosh/topics/antineoplastic

   - OSHA: http://www.osha.gov/SLTC/hazardousdrugs/recognition.html

In 2004, NIOSH issued an Alert titled, "Preventing Occupational Exposure to Antineoplastic and Other Hazardous Drugs in Health Care Settings" that details methods to eliminate or minimize occupational exposures [NIOSH 2004]. The document is an excellent resource for both management and employees to review to gain understanding in how to work safely with hazardous drugs.

RECOMMENDATIONS
(CONTINUED)

The results of additional monitoring during an actual procedure can assist in determining whether downgrading the level of personal protection equipment is appropriate.

REFERENCES

Bedford Laboratories [2009]. Cisplatin material safety data sheet. Bedford Laboratories, Bedford, Ohio. [http://www.bedfordlabs.com/BedfordLabsWeb/products/msdses/Cisplatin-1mgRev307.pdf]. Date accessed: December 2009.

IARC [2004]. IARC monographs on the evaluation of the carcinogenic risk of chemicals to humans. Lyons, France: World Health Organization, International Agency for Research on Cancer. [http://www.iarc.fr]. Date accessed: November 2009.

NCI [2009]. Cisplatin. Bethesda, Maryland. National Cancer Institute. [http://www.cancer.gov/cancertopics/druginfo/cisplatin]. Date accessed: November 2009.

NIOSH [2004]. NIOSH Alert: Preventing occupational exposure to antineoplastic and other hazardous drugs in health care settings. Cincinnati, OH: U.S. Department of Health and Human Services, Centers for Disease Control and Prevention, National Institute for Occupational Safety and Health, DHHS (NIOSH) Publication No. 2004-1193.

APPENDIX A: METHODS

Air samples were taken using Quick Take 30 high volume sample pumps (15 liters per minute) for GA samples and AirChek 2000 air sampling pumps (4 liters per minute) for PBZ samples. These samples were taken for the duration of the mock interperitoneal procedure (approximately 45 minutes). The sample media were analyzed for platinum (and then calculated as cisplatin) by ICP/MS with an LOD of 0.009 µg of cisplatin per sample and an LOQ of 0.029 µg of cisplatin per sample. The MDC of cisplatin in GA samples was 0.016 µg/m^3 based on a 576-liter air sample. The MDC of cisplatin in PBZ samples was 0.058 µg/m^3 based on a 157-liter air sample. The sampling method is an internal procedure developed by Bureau Veritas North America.

Wipe samples were taken using Alpha Texwipe swabs moistened with deionized water. A 10 cm x 10 cm square template was used to determine a 100 cm^2 sampling area. The sample media was analyzed for platinum (and then calculated as cisplatin) by ICP/MS with an LOD of 0.007 µg of cisplatin per sample and an LOQ of 0.031 µg of cisplatin per sample.

Cotton glove samples were worn beneath either Biogel latex gloves or nitrile chemotherapy protective gloves used by the hospital employees. NIOSH investigators, wearing sterile gloves, removed the cotton gloves from each employee after he or she had removed their outer chemotherapy protective gloves. Each pair of cotton gloves were analyzed for platinum (and then calculated as cisplatin) by ICP/MS. The LOD was 0.009 µg of cisplatin per sample, and the LOQ was 0.03 µg of cisplatin per sample.

APPENDIX B: OCCUPATIONAL EXPOSURE LIMITS AND HEALTH EFFECTS

In evaluating the hazards posed by workplace exposures, NIOSH investigators use both mandatory (legally enforceable) and recommended OELs for chemical, physical, and biological agents as a guide for making recommendations. OELs have been developed by Federal agencies and safety and health organizations to prevent the occurrence of adverse health effects from workplace exposures. Generally, OELs suggest levels of exposure that most employees may be exposed up to 10 hours per day, 40 hours per week for a working lifetime without experiencing adverse health effects. However, not all employees will be protected from adverse health effects even if their exposures are maintained below these levels. A small percentage may experience adverse health effects because of individual susceptibility, a preexisting medical condition, and/ or a hypersensitivity (allergy). In addition, some hazardous substances may act in combination with other workplace exposures, the general environment, or with medications or personal habits of the employee to produce health effects even if the occupational exposures are controlled at the level set by the exposure limit. Also, some substances can be absorbed by direct contact with the skin and mucous membranes in addition to being inhaled, which contributes to the individual's overall exposure.

Most OELs are expressed as a TWA exposure. A TWA refers to the average exposure during a normal 8- to 10-hour workday. Some chemical substances and physical agents have recommended STEL or ceiling values where health effects are caused by exposures over a short period. Unless otherwise noted, the STEL is a 15-minute TWA exposure that should not be exceeded at any time during a workday, and the ceiling limit is an exposure that should not be exceeded at any time.

In the United States, OELs have been established by Federal agencies, professional organizations, state and local governments, and other entities. Some OELs are legally enforceable limits, while others are recommendations. The U.S. Department of Labor OSHA PELs (29 CFR 1910 [general industry]; 29 CFR 1926 [construction industry]; and 29 CFR 1917 [maritime industry]) are legal limits enforceable in workplaces covered under the Occupational Safety and Health Act. NIOSH RELs are recommendations based on a critical review of the scientific and technical information available on a given hazard and the adequacy of methods to identify and control the hazard. NIOSH RELs can be found in the *NIOSH Pocket Guide to Chemical Hazards* [NIOSH 2005]. NIOSH also recommends different types of risk management practices (e.g., engineering controls, safe work practices, employee education/training, personal protective equipment, and exposure and medical monitoring) to minimize the risk of exposure and adverse health effects from these hazards. Other OELs that are commonly used and cited in the United States include the TLVs recommended by ACGIH, a professional organization, and the WEELs recommended by the American Industrial Hygiene Association, another professional organization. The TLVs and WEELs are developed by committee members of these associations from a review of the published, peer-reviewed literature. They are not consensus standards. ACGIH TLVs are considered voluntary exposure guidelines for use by industrial hygienists and others trained in this discipline "to assist in the control of health hazards" [ACGIH 2009]. WEELs have been established for some chemicals "when no other legal or authoritative limits exist" [AIHA 2009].

Outside the United States, OELs have been established by various agencies and organizations and include both legal and recommended limits. Since 2006, the Berufsgenossenschaftliches Institut für Arbeitsschutz (German Institute for Occupational Safety and Health) has maintained a database of international

OELs from European Union member states, Canada (Québec), Japan, Switzerland, and the United States available at http://www.dguv.de/bgia/en/gestis/limit_values/index.jsp. The database contains international limits for over 1250 hazardous substances and is updated annually.

Employers should understand that not all hazardous chemicals have specific OSHA PELs, and for some agents the legally enforceable and recommended limits may not reflect current health-based information. However, an employer is still required by OSHA to protect its employees from hazards even in the absence of a specific OSHA PEL. OSHA requires an employer to furnish employees a place of employment free from recognized hazards that cause or are likely to cause death or serious physical harm [Occupational Safety and Health Act of 1970 (Public Law 91–596, sec. 5(a)(1))]. Thus, NIOSH investigators encourage employers to make use of other OELs when making risk assessment and risk management decisions to best protect the health of their employees. NIOSH investigators also encourage the use of the traditional hierarchy of controls approach to eliminate or minimize identified workplace hazards. This includes, in order of preference, the use of: (1) substitution or elimination of the hazardous agent, (2) engineering controls (e.g , local exhaust ventilation, process enclosure, dilution ventilation), (3) administrative controls (e.g., limiting time of exposure, employee training, work practice changes, medical surveillance), and (4) personal protective equipment (e.g., respiratory protection, gloves, eye protection, hearing protection). Control banding, a qualitative risk assessment and risk management tool, is a complementary approach to protecting employee health that focuses resources on exposure controls by describing how a risk needs to be managed. Information on control banding is available at http://www.cdc.gov/niosh/topics/ctrlbanding/. This approach can be applied in situations where OELs have not been established or can be used to supplement the OELs, when available.

Cisplatin

Although OSHA and NIOSH have not established OELs for cisplatin, it has been categorized as a probable human carcinogen by IARC [IARC 2004]. Because of the potential carcinogenicity of cisplatin, exposures to cisplatin in pure form and in dilution should be controlled to the lowest achievable levels.

References

ACGIH [2009]. 2008 TLVs® and BEIs®: threshold limit values for chemical substances and physical agents and biological exposure indices. Cincinnati, OH: American Conference of Governmental Industrial Hygienists.

AIHA [2009]. AIHA 2008 Emergency response planning guidelines (ERPG) & workplace environmental exposure levels (WEEL) handbook. Fairfax, VA: American Industrial Hygiene Association.

CFR. Code of Federal Regulations. Washington, DC: U.S. Government Printing Office, Office of the Federal Register.

IARC [2004]. IARC monographs on the evaluation of the carcinogenic risk of chemicals to humans. Lyons, France: World Health Organization, International Agency for Research on Cancer. [http://www.iarc.fr]. Date accessed: November 2009.

NIOSH [2005]. NIOSH pocket guide to chemical hazards. Cincinnati, OH: U.S. Department of Health and Human Services, Centers for Disease Control and Prevention, National Institute for Occupational Safety and Health, DHHS (NIOSH) Publication No. 2005-149. [http://www.cdc.gov/niosh/npg/]. Date accessed: November 2009.

Appendix C: Tables

Table C1. Cisplatin sample results for general area and personal breathing zone air samples on May 11–12, 2009

Sample Location	Sample Description	Result (µg/m³)
	General Area Air Samples	
Inpatient Pharmacy	Senior pharmacy technician mixing cisplatin solution within chemical hood	ND*
Operating Room	Near head of operating table	ND*
Operating Room	At the head of operating table during mock procedure	ND*
Operating Room	At the foot of table during mock procedure	ND*
Operating Room	On instrument table during mock procedure	ND*
Outside	In hallway, adjacent to and just outside of operating room	ND*

* Not detected (concentration is below the MDC of 0.016 µg/m³, based on a 576-liter air sample)

Sample Location	Sample Description	Result (µg/m³)
	Personal Breathing Zone Air Samples	
Operating Room	Environmental Services manager sanitizing operating room after mock procedure	ND†
Operating Room	Registered nurse preparing and spiking cisplatin IV bag	ND†
Operating Room	Surgical technician assisting physician	ND†
Operating Room	Physician administering and manipulating the cisplatin solution within the metal pan	ND†
Sterile Processing	Sterile Processing manager sterilizing equipment used in mock procedure	ND†

† Not detected (concentration is below the MDC of 0.058 µg/m³, based on a 157-liter air sample)

Table C2. Cisplatin wipe sample results using Alpha TexWipe swabs on May 11–12, 2009

Sample Location	Sample Description	Result (µg/sample)*
Inpatient Pharmacy	Surface of chemotherapy mixing hood after cisplatin solution was prepared	ND†
Operating Room *(before mock interperitoneal procedure)*	On floor away from cisplatin	ND†
	On floor nearside to cisplatin	ND†
	On floor, at head of operating table	ND†
	Hand wipe from registered nurse	ND‡
	Hand wipe from Environmental Services manager	ND‡
Operating Room *(after mock interperitoneal procedure but before sanitization)*	On floor away from cisplatin	ND†
	On floor nearside to cisplatin	0.08
	On floor, at head of operating table	ND†
Sterile Processing	Surface of stainless steel decontamination sink (sink contained 10% bleach solution)	ND†
	Surface of stainless steel rinse sink	ND†
	On cart used to transport surgical instruments from operating room to sterile processing	ND†
Operating Room *(after sanitization)*	On floor away from cisplatin	ND†
	On floor nearside from cisplatin	ND†
	On floor at head of operating table	ND†

* A 10 cm x 10 cm square disposable template was used to define the sampling area.
† ND = not detected (below the LOD of 0.007 µg of cisplatin per sample)
‡ The hand wipe samples were collected by swabbing both hands of the employee with an Alpha TexWipe moistened with deionized water. A disposable template was not used for these samples.

Table C3. Cisplatin sample results for cotton glove samples on May 11–12, 2009

Sample Location	Outer Glove	Sample Description	Result (µg/sample)
Inpatient Pharmacy	Nitrile chemotherapy gloves	Senior pharmacy technician mixing cisplatin solution in chemical hood	ND†
Operating Room	Biogel	Physician adding and manipulating cisplatin in the metal pan	ND†
Operating Room	Nitrile chemotherapy gloves	Registered nurse spiking cisplatin intravenous bag and assisting in the mock procedure	ND†
Operating Room	Biogel	Surgical technician assisting physician during mock procedure	ND†
Sterile Processing	Nitrile chemotherapy gloves	Manager sterilizing equipment used in mock procedure	ND†
Environmental Services	Nitrile chemotherapy gloves	Manager cleaning/sanitizing room after mock procedure	ND†
Environmental Services	Nitrile chemotherapy gloves	Manager cleaning/sanitizing room after mock procedure	ND†

* Each sample consisted of a pair of cotton gloves worn by the employee beneath their outer chemotherapy-approved gloves.
† ND = not detected (below the LOD of 0.009 µg of cisplatin per sample)

This page intentionally left blank.

Acknowledgments and Availability of Report

The Hazard Evaluations and Technical Assistance Branch (HETAB) of the National Institute for Occupational Safety and Health (NIOSH) conducts field investigations of possible health hazards in the workplace. These investigations are conducted under the authority of Section 20(a)(6) of the Occupational Safety and Health (OSH) Act of 1970, 29 U.S.C. 669(a)(6) which authorizes the Secretary of Health and Human Services, following a written request from any employer or authorized representative of employees, to determine whether any substance normally found in the place of employment has potentially toxic effects in such concentrations as used or found. HETAB also provides, upon request, technical and consultative assistance to federal, state, and local agencies; labor; industry; and other groups or individuals to control occupational health hazards and to prevent related trauma and disease.

The findings and conclusions in this report are those of the authors and do not necessarily represent the views of NIOSH. Mention of any company or product does not constitute endorsement by NIOSH. In addition, citations to websites external to NIOSH do not constitute NIOSH endorsement of the sponsoring organizations or their programs or products. Furthermore, NIOSH is not responsible for the content of these websites. All Web addresses referenced in this document were accessible as of the publication date.

This report was prepared by James Couch and Gregory Burr of HETAB, Division of Surveillance, Hazard Evaluations and Field Studies. Health communication assistance was provided by Stefanie Evans. Editorial assistance was provided by Ellen Galloway. Desktop publishing was performed by Robin Smith.

Copies of this report have been sent to employee and management representatives at University Medical Center, the state health department, and the Occupational Safety and Health Administration Regional Office. This report is not copyrighted and may be freely reproduced. The report may be viewed and printed at http://www.cdc.gov/niosh/hhe/. Copies may be purchased from the National Technical Information Service at 5825 Port Royal Road, Springfield, Virginia 22161.

NIOSH [2010]. Health hazard evaluation report: evaluation of exposures to healthcare personnel from cisplatin during a mock interperitoneal operation, Las Vegas, NV. By Couch J and Burr G. Cincinnati, OH: U.S. Department of Health and Human Services, Centers for Disease Control and Prevention, National Institute for Occupational Safety and Health, NIOSH HETA No. 2009-0121-3106.

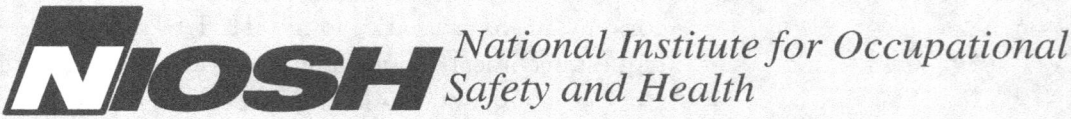
National Institute for Occupational Safety and Health

Delivering on the Nation's promise: Safety and health at work for all people through research and prevention.

To receive NIOSH documents or information about occupational safety and health topics, contact NIOSH at:

1-800-CDC-INFO (1-800-232-4636)

TTY: 1-888-232-6348

E-mail: cdcinfo@cdc.gov

or visit the NIOSH web site at: **www.cdc.gov/niosh**.

For a monthly update on news at NIOSH, subscribe to NIOSH eNews by visiting **www.cdc.gov/niosh/eNews**.

SAFER • HEALTHIER • PEOPLE™

www.ingramcontent.com/pod-product-compliance
Lightning Source LLC
Chambersburg PA
CBHW080941290526
45795CB00007BA/2852